BACK ORGANIC GARDENING:

Mastering Ways to Grow your Own Food.

©2017 William Canterbury

http://www.FunHappyLives.com

© Copyright 2017 by CiJiRO Publishing- All rights reserved.

This document is geared toward providing exact and reliable information in regard to the topic and issue covered. The publication is sold with the idea that the publisher is not required to render accounting, officially permitted, or otherwise, qualified services. If advice is necessary, legal or professional, a practiced individual in the profession should be ordered.

- From a Declaration of Principles which was accepted and approved equally by a Committee of the American Bar Association and a Committee of Publishers and Associations.

In no way is it legal to reproduce, duplicate, or transmit any part of this document in either electronic means or in printed format. Recording of this publication is strictly prohibited and any storage of this document is not allowed unless with written permission from the publisher. All rights reserved.

The information provided herein is stated to be truthful and consistent, in that any liability, in terms of inattention or otherwise, by any usage or abuse of any policies, processes, or directions contained within is the solitary and utter responsibility of the recipient reader. Under no circumstances will any legal responsibility or blame be held against the publisher for any reparation, damages, or monetary loss due to the information herein, either directly or indirectly.

Respective authors own all copyrights not held by the publisher.

The information herein is offered for informational purposes solely, and is universal as so. The presentation of the information is without contract or any type of guarantee assurance.

The trademarks that are used are without any consent, and the publication of the trademark is without permission or backing by the trademark owner. All trademarks and brands within this book are for clarifying purposes only and are the owned by the owners themselves, not affiliated with this document.

Introduction

What is the Back to Eden Style of Gardening?
In the same size as a double-bed you can feed your family every day with organically grown fresh vegetables in just a few months. If you have some property in your back yard or you live in the city and have only a single bed size to spare, it is easier than you think.

Today people are able to get all the required to start a food garden that will fit on the balcony of an apartment. One can purchase containers that can drain the soil as required, or one could even test the quality of the soil created to very precise measurements.

For less than $50 you can purchase potting soil and containers, with a few dollars spent on seeds you, will be able to feed your family after a few months. You will get a lot more than good health because of the improved efficiency of your metabolism and how your body detoxifies itself. You will also hopefully discover that 'connection' which created our bodies millions of year ago.

Our digestion is not built to digest unprocessed organic foods, even 100 years after the invention of junk and processed foods we still see no adaptation to our ability to withstand these toxic onslaughts that go through us every day. When we put our hands in the soil there is a possibility that we can find that 'connection' with our creator.

There is a reciprocity that you can feel, even though it may take a few months of eating organic foods, you will feel that there is more than just the growing of a carrot or potato in your food garden. However good or bad it might feel to be see something grow that you were responsible for, you will know deep inside that you are making that 'connection.'

Whether you believe in the bible or not, the metaphor of the Garden of Eden is something we can scientifically prove. Any contemporary dietitian or nutritionist will tell you to stay away from processed foods and rather eat organic foods that are without toxins.

The Paleo Diet based on the "The Primal Blueprint" written by Mark Sisson has been extensively researched proving that our genetic ability to handle processed food is not getting any better. The highly processed foods we eat every day how now shown to cause diseases Cancer and Diabetes that increase every year at an alarming rate with diabetes now the fastest growing disease on the planet.

The only solution is to do something about it so we can 'connect' to the reason why the creator put us here in the first place. Our genetic predisposition when eating correctly gives us increased efficiency when consuming organic foods and health as a result becomes self-evident.

The basic foundation on which our bodies started to evolve over millions of years is built on eating foods that our bodies are originally designed to eat. The same can be applied to treating a new auto-mobile exactly as specified by the manufacturer.

A car will last a lot longer if treated correctly, a healthy auto-mobile will outlive any unhealthy badly treated auto-mobile. If the car is treated correctly as indicated by the manufacturers it will last a lot longer than not caring for it.

If we follow the directions as indicated by our creator based on solid research done on the best foods to eat. With all the state of the art science we have available we still cannot find a better way to feed ourselves than by eating organically grown foods as indicated by our creator. Science has still not found a better way to feed ourselves.

Creating a food garden should be the topic of conversation at all dinner tables around the world. It starts with education and knowing that this 'connection' is possible by simply feeding oneself in the most efficient way because we are what we eat

Thank you for purchasing my book. It is my sincere hope it will answer your question on title

Contents

Introduction 5

Chapter 1. Comparison to Other Gardening Styles 13

Chapter 2. The Covering 23

Chapter 3. Choosing the Garden Location..41

Chapter 4. Creating the Garden ...45

Chapter 5. Planting the Garden ...50

Conclusion 61

Chapter 1. Comparison to Other Gardening Styles

Conventional Garden

A conventional garden is how many people start. Most simply set aside a portion of their yard that has adequate sun, rototill it up, and start planting. This has the advantage of being an extremely cheap way to garden (if you don't count the rotor tiller cost). For nutrients, compost or manure can be spread on top and tilled in. Watering will generally be done by hand. The bare soil will encourage weeds, so time must be spent pulling them.

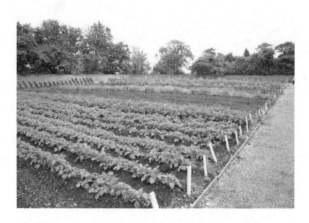

As you can see, this type of garden has a low upfront cost (unlike raised beds) but requires more labor to maintain later on. And of course the soil will compact and harden through the year. Every spring the soil will need to be tilled or spaded to loosen it prior to planting. Care must then be taken not to step on and compact the soil as much as possible, particularly around the plants. The bare dirt will turn to mud when wet so you will want to stay out of the garden until it dries.

Tilling is one of the major drawbacks in the conventional garden style. You either have to spend hours of hard labor with a shovel or spade loosening the soil, or you have to spend hundreds of dollars on a rotor tiller. Also rotor tillers generally only loosen the soil for approximately 6 inches down, when plant roots can go much deeper.

Raised Beds

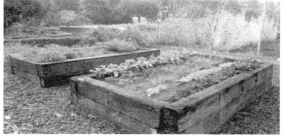

I first started gardening with raised beds and they did well, but quickly got expensive. When I first started making them, I filled them with a growing soil mix delivered from a nursery. The plants loved it, but at $40 a yard I was having a real problem justifying the price. Later I started hauling in composted horse manure from my mother-in-law's farm. This was free, but did bring in weeds, a lot of them. However, the easy access to the raised beds made it fairly simple to keep the weeds under control.

Obviously, the greatest benefit to raised beds is that you can start with good growing soil from the beginning and not have to build it up. This allows you to plant quite intensively (like with square foot gardening). I was able to produce extraordinary amounts of produce at first, but noticed that my yields diminished every following year as the nutrients were absorbed out of the soil. Also the soil in the beds would keep settling. What had been level with the top of the boards in spring would be 2 inches below them in the fall.

As I continued building raised beds over the years I could no longer afford the growing mix and switched to the compost horse manure. That saved me the money I had been spending on soil, but still left the cost for the lumber. A single one of my 4' x 12' raised beds made out of untreated 2x12" lumber from Home Depot cost me $50.

Another major problem was watering. I quickly realized that raised beds are very inefficient for watering as the water quickly runs through them. I live in a very dry climate and soon realized that watering by hand was not practical. So then I had to invest in a drip irrigation system. Eventually, I had my entire garden set up so I could just come out and turn my outdoor faucet on, and every single raised bed would be watered. Unfortunately, this was also expensive. Every raised bed cost about $25 for the drip emitters, tubing, and connectors it required.

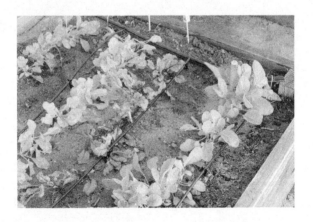

Then there were the problems I had with soil compaction. The first year the beds were freshly made and the soil was all nice and loose. Needless to say, the plants loved that. But every year following that, I had to spade the soil to loosen it prior to planting, and that quickly got on my nerves.

But the real problem I had with raided beds was the cost. Every new 4'x12' bed I built was costing me nearly $150 using the growing mix or $75 if I used the composted manure. I had wanted to make up to 20 of the raised beds, but could just not justify the cost. Fortunately it was at that time that I first saw the Back to Eden film and realized there was a better way.

Back to Eden Style

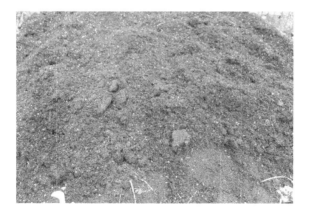

This is essentially the same as a conventional style, but with 4 to 6 inches of organic covering (acting as mulch) on the soil year around. That simple addition fixes nearly all the negatives of the other styles.

*The covering prevents the sun from hitting the soil and killing the microbes.

*It dramatically reduces the soil compaction, and therefore, need to till.

*It dramatically reduces water evaporation from the soil and therefore requires a fraction of the watering needed by the raised bed and conventional styles.

*It dramatically suppresses weed growth.

*The covering gradually decomposes and in turn, fertilizes the soil.

*It is very cheap, as most covering materials can be had for free.

*The covering allows you to access the garden cleanly, even when it is muddy outside.

One of the common misconceptions about the back to Eden style of gardening is that all that carbon rich material touching on the soil will rob the nitrogen out of the soil during the decomposition process. Nothing could be farther from the truth. Only the top 1/16th of an inch of the soil is in contact with the covering and could ever possibly be affected. As long as the covering is simply lying on top of the soil, and not mixed in with it, you will be fine.

Peat moss used in this example

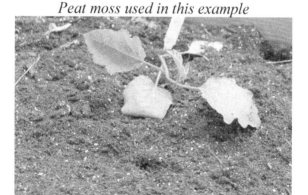

When I first watched the Back to Eden film, I knew this was something I wanted to do. I disassembled some of my older raised beds and spread the soil out evenly. Then I had my first load of wood chips from a tree trimming company delivered and covered that ground with 6 inches worth. Unfortunately, that following spring I became busy with work commitments, and had a much smaller garden than I had planned.

I decided to just plant in my regular raised beds that year, and leave the Back to Eden section for the following year. However I noticed several "volunteer" squash plants come through the wood chips from the area I had previously raised squash. As I had also planted the same variety of squash that year in my remaining raised beds, I figured this would be a good comparison to see which system grew better plants.

Not surprisingly, the squash plants growing out of the wood chips quickly surpassed the ones in my raised beds. At their peak, they were nearly 5 feet wide and some 3 feet high. Another glaring difference I noticed was how they handled high temperatures. When temperatures reached into the upper 90's, the squash plants in my raised beds would be badly wilted, despite being watered daily. However the squash plants in the wood chips displayed no ill effects. In fact, the wood chips did such a good job of insulating the soil that I only watered those particular plants approximately 5 times through the whole summer, and it was debatable if they even needed that much watering. I quickly realized that there was something to this style of gardening.

Chapter 2. The Covering

Hopefully by now I have convinced you to give the Back to Eden style of gardening a try. Therefore your next step is to locate material that you can use to cover your soil.

Woodchips

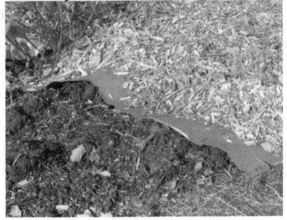

Woodchips were the covering of choice used in the Back to Eden film. These can generally be obtained from tree trimming companies for free. You may have to call several companies before you can find somebody to bring them to you. When I first started calling around to get woodchips delivered I had fits at first.

As it turns out, there is mainly just one tree trimming company in the area, and they told me they would "put me on their list". Several weeks went by and still no woodchips. Finally somebody suggested I call the electric company and find out who clears the right of ways for the power lines. The nice lady at the electric company gave me the cell phone number of the foreman of the crew that did that for them, and he said he would see what he could do. And about a week later, sure enough, I had my first woodchips delivered.

However, that's when I discovered there is huge disparity in the size of "wood chips". The woodchips I had seen in the film were small, and most pieces were between one half and 1 inch in diameter and that's what I was expecting to get. Instead, what I got was what I would describe as broken up sticks. It was mostly ground-up limbs and twigs, and the average "woodchip" was half of a inch wide and 4 inches long.

Amazingly, many sticks had come through their chipper relatively unscathed and I had many that were 18 inches long, as you can see in the picture below.

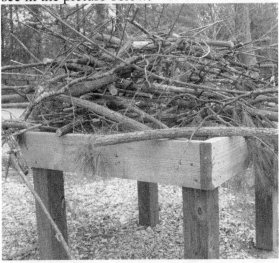

As a result of so many long sticks in the pile, it was a terrible a pain to shovel and move the wood chips. Then once I had it spread out I discovered it did a poor job of keeping moisture in the soil. Basically, the larger the wood chips the bigger the gaps between them, and therefore, the worse they were as mulch. Also, because they dried out so easily they also decomposed extremely slowly.

When I checked around, I found out many people commenting that the wood chips that were delivered to them did not look like the ones show in the Back to Eden film. A big reason for that is the ones in the film were processed with a tub grinder, which grinds the chips much smaller than the machines the tree trimming companies use. Also, there may be a disparity in wood chip size between different tree trimming companies. After several years I was finally able to get woodchips delivered from the main tree trimming company I mentioned earlier, and their shredder produced much smaller woodchips than the one used by the electric company's crew.

Eventually, I hired the tree trimming company to remove an 85 foot elm tree in my front yard and leave me all the woodchips from it, which they were happy to do. During that time I become friends with several of the trimming crew, and can get woodchips delivered whenever I want now days.

One thing that has surprised me is how fast the woodchips will decompose even if left in a pile. Some of the wood chip piles left over from my elm tree removal were left untouched for six months before I got around to using them. Once I dug into them I was amazed at how advanced the decomposition already was. They break down fast if kept moist. Incidentally, when it comes to moving woodchips I have found the easiest method is to use a pitchfork. It will slice into the piles so much easier than a shovel will. Moving a huge pile of woodchips is a time-consuming and laborious task, but I found my speed increased about 50% when I switched to using a pitchfork instead of shovel.

Generally, I will use the pitchfork to fill up my wheelbarrow and then go dump it were it is needed. However, people have also told me they have had great results moving the woodchips around using 55 gallon barrels and a dolly.

So the first thing to do is start calling the tree service companies in your area and asking for them to drop off their woodchips at your location. They will generally be happy to do so as long as it is convenient for them. Don't expect them to drive 10 miles out in the country just to give you their woodchips for free. If they seem to balk at the distance, perhaps you can offer to pay for their gas.

You will be quite surprised at how much woodchips it can take to cover your garden 4 to 6 inches deep. I have had wood chip piles the size of a car delivered to me only to find that it was barely enough to cover about 350 square feet. Also, the woodchips will settle very quickly once you've had a few rain showers, and you may realize you have much thinner of a covering than you thought you had.

If you have trouble getting wood chips from the tree service companies try putting a request up on www.freecycle.org. There is a great website that will put you on a national woodchip list called www.abouttrees.com. They will add you to their database to connect people wanting wood chips to companies that need to get rid of them.

Drive around your neighborhood just after a big storm or when they are doing road work and look for the tree service trucks. Tell them that you live around the corner and they can dump the woodchips in your driveway. This will save them time and gas, so they are usually up for it.

Wood chips are the most popular form of covering for Back to Eden style gardens because you can get large, if not enormous, quantities delivered to you for free. However, some people have reported great difficulty in getting woodchips and so may need to look at other alternatives for covering material.

Sawdust

It was several years from when I first had my rather disappointing woodchips delivered from the electric company to the time I was able to start getting good quality woodchips from the tree trimming company. The electric company ended up dropping off two loads of woodchips for me to use the first year before I told them that I had enough. The truth was, of course, that I was tired of them delivering me piles of small sticks instead of woodchips.

So I started looking around for any other types of alternatives and discovered sawdust. As it turns out, a friend of my mother's rented out part of her land to be used by a man who cut and sold firewood for a living. He had quite the operation, with huge piles of logs and multiple wood splitters. The entire area was covered with a thick layer of sawdust from chainsaws. Some of the sawdust had been lying on the ground for several years and had already turned a dark brown color. Periodically, they would use a bobcat to clear the sawdust out of the area and push it into large piles.

I researched the concept of using sawdust as mulch and found many success stories. The only caveats I found were to avoid fresh sawdust that still had turpentine in it, and to avoid very fine sawdust, as it would not let water penetrate. Therefore, I reasoned that this aged sawdust made by chainsaws should be perfectly fine for use as mulch, and indeed it was.

I made multiple trips bringing sawdust from those piles and spreading it upon my garden. The dark brown colored sawdust looked fantastic spread across the garden and was great mulch. It held moisture in the soil very well, and broke down very quickly into compost. To be honest, I think I actually prefer aged sawdust as a covering instead of woodchips, but it sure is nice to have the 12+ cubic yards worth of woodchips delivered right to me, versus having to haul the sawdust myself over many trips.

However, if you are having trouble getting woodchips, try checking into sawdust as a covering. I have been told about a local sawmill that will fill your entire pickup truck bed with sawdust and only charges five dollars a load. Perhaps you have something similar near you. Again, try and get the oldest and darkest sawdust you can find.

Straw, Hay, and Leaves
Many people have wondered about mulching with hay, straw or leaves. The short answer is that all of these are perfectly acceptable as a covering. Arguably, it was probably *Ruth Stout* who first popularized the concept of a year-round covering for the soil back in the '50s and '60s. Her system involved laying down a thick layer of straw as a mulch to greatly reduce watering and weeding, and she wrote several popular books on the subject. Although I think woodchips and sawdust are much better alternatives for covering, you may be in a situation where those are not readily available and you require a substitute.

Although I have never used anything other than woodchips and sawdust for my garden personally, I did try to do a composting experiment with hay bales last year. Just as Paul has done in the Back to Eden film, I have turned my chicken run into my composting system. My chickens have approximately 300 square feet worth of run with 6 foot high fencing, and for years now I have been throwing all my compostable items into that chicken run. Just like in the film, the chickens will happily eat what they want, then mix in and stir around the remainder as it becomes compost. Each fall I will also rake up and deposit all the leaves from my property into the chicken run, where they would quickly become compost.

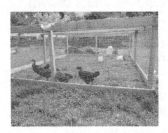

Eventually, I designed a routine where every fall I would load up the chicken run with several feet worth of my leaves and whatever other types of organic material I could find. By the following fall it had become about a 6 inch layer of compost that I would then spread across my garden.

The first year I loaded up my chicken run with a load of the "shredded sticks" the electric company guys dropped off. They composted okay, but some of the pieces were not completely decomposed when it was time to spread them out the following year. The second year I put in a foot worth of the aged sawdust. That decomposed absolutely perfectly and had completely turned into compost by the next year.

But the third-year I wanted to try something different and so decided to try composting hay bales. We had an unusually wet summer that year, and a lot of hay had been spoiled. I put an ad on craigslist asking for spoiled hay for composting and quickly collected some 50 bales worth. I spread them out across my chicken run and arranged them so the straw was orientated vertically, in hopes that water could more easily penetrate the bales. That was a year ago, and I think I can safely say I will never do that again. About one third of the straw still has not decomposed and has turned into a wet, matted mass. Looks like I'm going to have to give it another year. Still the experience showed me that it's not hard to find free spoiled hay on craigslist if you need it. And of course, you could purchase fresh bales of hay and straw at any farm supply store.

However, new bales are not cheap, so if you need to cover a large area you had best try and locate spoiled bales that can be had for free. I was not concerned about grass or weed seeds in the bales of hay I obtained because I figured the chickens would eat them, especially once they sprouted. However, the hay bales that I did obtain were absolutely loaded with seeds, and I would certainly not have wanted to apply them directly to my garden. Hay will have by far the most seeds in it, but even straw will have at least a small amount in my experience.

However, if you do use straw or hay for your covering, make ABSOLUTLY SURE that the hay has never been sprayed with herbicides, as some of them can survive being composted and can ruin your garden for years. These types of persistent herbicides were designed specifically for use in farmer's fields and can pass through the livestock without being absorbed. These herbicides also readily survive composting. Once in the soil, they can remain active for up to 7 years, and are harmful to garden plants at one part per million.

A quick Google search will show you many heartbreaking stories of gardeners who have been sabotaged by these types of herbicides, as well as compost companies that have been forced to shut down after these herbicides found their way into the compost. I did not realize these type of persistent herbicides even existed until after the hay had already been placed into my chicken run so I will have to be careful were I apply this compost just to be on the safe side.

Also, for the same reason, I would be very wary of using grass clippings as a cover unless you are certain they have not been sprayed with herbicides. That is a shame really, as I see so many landscaping company trucks driving around my town with huge loads of grass clippings they are hauling away. I have often toyed with the idea of asking them to dump the clippings at my house and use them for composting in my chicken run. Grass clippings breakdown extremely quickly into compost and would be an excellent resource. But I just don't want to take the risk of my garden getting contaminated by herbicides.

Leaves, fortunately, do not carry the risk of being contaminated with herbicides. If you can locate a sufficient quantity they are reported to do a decent job as mulch. Wetting them thoroughly after covering the soil will result in them forming a sort of matted layer, and will help prevent the leaves being blown away

Regardless of the type of covering you choose to use, it is highly advisable to put down newspaper or cardboard over the garden area before applying the covering. This will drastically reduce if not outright eliminate weeds and grass from growing up through the covering.

Several people have asked if it is necessary to till up the soil before applying the covering. Personally I would not bother unless the soil is currently as hard as a rock and you will be planting right away. Once the covering is applied, the soil will begin to loosen and will continue to do so as the months go by. Ideally, the covering will be applied in the fall and the first planting will take place the following spring.

Another common concern is that nitrogen will be robbed from the soil and used to decompose the carbon material in the organic covering. This is not a problem if the covering is simply lying on top, as only perhaps the top 1/16 of an inch of the soil will be in contact with the carbon material.

You would not want to mix in or till the covering material into the soil though, as that would rob the soil of nitrogen for about a year as the organisms break down the carbon material. You would probably have some fantastic soil by the second year though.

Chapter 3. Choosing the Garden Location

Some of you may have a teeny lot with only one possible spot to garden. Others may have a lot of land and have many possible places for a garden. What many people don't realize is where you put your garden plays a large role in your success.

Convenience

The position of the garden should first and foremost be chosen for convenience. After all, a vegetable garden is for your enjoyment. The "Back to Eden" style of gardening requires much less maintenance than a regular garden, but you still will need to harvest regularly. Remember this mantra: out of sight, out of mind.

Sunlight

Another thing to consider when choosing a garden location is how much sun that spot gets. Typically, vegetables need at least 6 hours of sun, though 8 or more hours is better. This is probably the second largest consideration when making a garden. Everything else can be fixed to some degree, but not the sun. Generally speaking, you want your plants to receive the most sun they can possibly get, as this has a direct correlation to their growth and health.

Drainage
Plants can't grow in waterlogged soil. If the location of a vegetable garden is at the bottom of a hill or in an indentation in the ground, it will have a hard time drying out and the plants will suffer.

Wind
High winds can wreak havoc on a garden in a matter of minutes. Most of the time, high winds will come from a single direction on your property. Try and place your garden where it can be at least somewhat protected from the prevailing winds.

Soil
Soil is not as much a factor in where to place a garden as you might think The one thing you definitely want to avoid is having a lot of rocks in your soil. This was a major problem for me, as my front yard has the worst soil I've ever seen mixed in with about 50% rocks by volume. By contrast, my backyard has very few rocks and much better soil. It is amazing how much of a difference just 50 feet can make.

Water

this is still a necessary consideration, even with a "Back to Eden" style garden. Though this style requires much less water than a conventional garden, it still will need some watering in my experience.

At a bare minimum, you will probably need to water right after the initial planting in the spring. Paul's garden in the film does not require watering through the summer, but I have not been able to duplicate that entirely at my location. I still need to water approximately 10 times throughout the summer here in the southwest part of the country. Therefore, the garden does need to be in proximity to a water source.

Chapter 4. Creating the Garden

Once you have determined where the garden will be, the next step is applying the weed barrier, any compost, and of course the covering.

Weed barrier
applying a weed barrier over the soil will dramatically decrease the amount of weeds you will have to deal with, particularly in the first year, when they tend to be the worst. Since you will have to plant through this, it needs to be a biodegradable material, such as cardboard or newspaper.

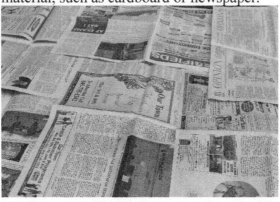

You will want a single layer of cardboard or four layers of newspaper at a minimum. Personally, I prefer double that. Remember, you can't come back later and redo this, so it's best to do it right the first time. You can acquire cardboard boxes fairly easily by inquiring at local stores and businesses. Also, see if your community as a location for recycling cardboard. Newspaper can often be had in large amounts simply by asking your local newspaper company for any unsold or old newspapers. Also, many people have reported acquiring rolls of newsprint from them, some 4 feet wide, that they simply unrolled across the garden.

Obviously, you want to apply this weed barrier on a day with no wind. It is easiest to put down a little at a time and dump some compost or covering on it to hold it down as you go. This barrier will have decomposed by the end of the first growing season, but after that you should have very little problem with weeds.

Compost
you may not need to apply this if your soil is already very good. But for most people, applying several inches of compost over the garden will really help and I recommend it. You will probably require a large amount of compost to cover an entire garden, and it will be very expensive if you are buying bagged compost. So what I like to do is use composted manure.

This can generally be had for free with a little searching. A single horse can put out 50 pounds of manure a day, and the owner is usually extremely happy to get rid of it. That being said, I somewhat prefer cow manure to horse manure, as it has fewer viable weed seeds. Many people who keep livestock will have piles of manure that have been aged a year or more, and are perfect for use in the garden.

Simply spread this over the weed barrier several inches thick and it will provide the nutrients the plants can use for the next few years. By then the initial covering will be well on its way to being compost itself and can begin fertilizing the plants.

The Covering
Finally you can apply the covering you have chosen over the garden. Getting the depth right can be a little tricky. Generally you want between four and 6 inches of covering. Any more than 6 inches and it gets too difficult to move it aside for planting. However, generally there will be some settling of the material for several weeks after you apply it.

Woodchips, in particular, are quite bad at this. I can apply 8 inches of woodchips across my garden and have it settle down to 5 inches or even less within a few weeks. How thick it needs to be will also depend on the size of the covering material. For example, large, chunky woodchips will have many air passageways between them that will let the ground moisture escape. Therefore, it will need to be applied in a thicker layer than say, smaller sized woodchips, or sawdust would need to be applied.

I would advise you to start with a minimum amount of covering at first, and add more later on if needed. After all, it is much easier to add additional covering than it is to remove excess covering.

And that is all there is to it. Now you have your Back to Eden garden ready and all that's left is to start planting!!

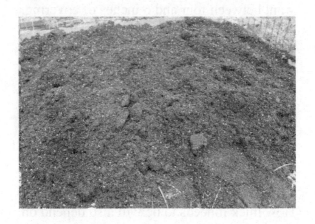

Chapter 5. Planting the Garden

Okay, now you have your covering spread out across your gardening and we are ready to get to the fun part, planting the garden. This is no different than planting in a conventional garden except you will have to move the covering aside to access the soil.

What I use is two metal stakes connected by a long piece of twine that I use to arrange my rows with. I place the stakes apart at both ends of the garden and pound them into the ground. Then I follow along under the twine between them, raking the covering aside until the soil is exposed to view. Then I simply move both stakes over 3 feet, pound them in again, and repeat the process. This gives me neat, orderly, straight rows throughout my garden. Then I will simply go back and plant in the uncovered soil in each row.

If I am putting in transplants, I will move the covering back up around the stem as I plant. If I am planting seeds I will leave the soil bare for now, as I have learned that some seeds resent having to grow through even the slightest layer of covering. I will come back to spread the covering around them in a few weeks once they are at least a few inches tall. Make sure you have raked away the covering from the rows enough that the covering will not slide down and smother the sprouting plants. This has been a problem for me in the past, particularly during high winds. As the plants continue to grow, you will simply continue to move back the covering against them until eventually it will be as thick as it was before you raked it away.

Potatoes are abnormal in that they will happily grow through up though 12 inches of woodchips, as has been in my experience. So they will get buried quite deeply with covering immediately after planting.

Plant spacing is generally the same in the Back to Eden garden as it would be in a conventional garden. However, as the system really starts to kick in over the years, you may need to increase the spacing over time.

Because the soil will be kept so incredibly loose and fluffy, the plant's root systems will grow far larger than they normally would. This will, of course, result in much larger plants. In fact, *Paul Gautschi* from the Back to Eden film has reported that since he covered his orchard with woodchips, he now has to plant new trees at double the recommended spacing, because they will grow double the size they were supposed to. What a wonderful problem to have.

Watering
Obviously, with a thick layer of mulch across your garden, your garden's watering needs will be drastically reduced. In the Back to Eden film, Paul does not have to water his garden, other than when he first plants. In the extremely dry climate where I am located I have had to water, but it is indeed a fraction of what it used to need. The most critical time is the first few weeks after you have planted the garden. At this time the seeds are still sprouting and all the vegetation is so low you cannot replace the covering without smothering them.

So I take care to keep the soil moist during this time. However, once the plants have grown enough that I can have them covered with the 4 to 6 inches of mulch, my watering went way down to perhaps every second or third week. By about the middle of July the plant's roots were developed enough that I could stop watering for the rest of the season.

Obviously, how much you will have to water your garden using the Back to Eden style will depend greatly upon your climate as well as the quality of your covering.

Fertilizing

I have come across people who have been disgruntled after trying the Back to Eden style of gardening. The most common complaint, by far, is that their plants were nothing like the large, vigorous ones they saw in the film. However, many of these people were first-time gardeners, and/or had planted into soil that was marginal at best. You cannot simply throw the covering on the ground and walk away expecting to return to magnificent yields.

Some people have the perception that fertilizer was not required because the covering would provide it as it decomposed. This is indeed true over time, but it is important to note that this will take years. My personal observations have been that approximately 1 to 2 inches of the covering decomposes each year. But that may only correlate to as little as a quarter of an inch of compost being created yearly. As the years go past, the soil will indeed become richer and richer, and after a decade or so it will be incredible. But for those just starting out, and who have marginal soil, some type of fertilizer is highly recommended.

The best time to apply the fertilizer is before the covering is applied. Ideally, you would lay down your newspaper or cardboard for weed control, followed by 2 to 3 inches of composted manure, followed by 4 to 6 inches of your covering material.

That should provide enough fertilizer to keep the garden going for several years at least, and after, that the initial covering will be well on its way towards becoming compost. As the covering becomes thin, more organic material would be added to the cover to bring it back to the desired 4 to 6 inches of thickness. This will result in your soil being constantly fed with compost until it eventually reaches the level of richness seen in the film.

If the covering has already been applied, you can still apply the composted manure fairly effectively. Just spread it across the covering and let the rains wash it down to the soil. This would also cause the covering to decompose even faster. The only downside would be that weeds will readily grow from the manure if it is not under the covering.

Weeds
having a thick layer of covering across the soil has drastically reduced the amount of weeds in my garden. However, I still have a problem with Bindweed at my place, as it actually seems to prefer growing in mulch. In fact, when I was getting sawdust for my covering years ago, I observed Bindweed growing on the piles of sawdust that had roots reaching over 2 feet down into the piles. Needless to say, my 6 inches of covering doesn't even slow it down. However, at least one upside to this is that the Bindweed is actually my chicken's absolute favorite food. So whenever I see some I will pull it up and toss it into my chicken run.

I have also heard that crabgrass as well as several other types of weeds will readily grow through coverings. Honestly, the best prevention against weeds is to put down a thick layer of newspaper or cardboard prior to applying your covering, as that will make a huge difference. However, even with my Bindweed problem, my garden is, in fact, remarkably weed free since I switched to using the Back to Eden style of gardening. And that alone has saved me many hours of labor through the summer months.

One of the many benefits to the Back to Eden style of gardening is that the covering will keep the soil soft and loose. This, of course, will cause the plant roots to grow through the soil much easier. This also means that whatever weeds do manage to grow through the covering will be extremely easy to pull up. In fact, you should be able to pull them up using only two fingers.

Let me take this time to highly recommend you to own chickens, as they are wonderful companions to the garden. Ever since I got chickens I have not seen weeds as something negative, but rather as free chicken food. Also, there will be a tremendous amount of waste that comes out of the garden that can be fed to the chickens. Did the squash get to the size of a baseball bat overnight?

No problem, simply chop it up and give it to the chickens. Same with disfigured tomatoes or any other damaged vegetables. In exchange, the chickens give me eggs, a large amount of compost (both from the run and inside their coop), and a tremendous amount of enjoyment from watching their antics. It really is a perfect symbiotic relationship.

Pest and Disease
Now I'm certainly not going to claim that the Back to Eden style of gardening will miraculously eliminate your problems with pest and disease. However, I think I can safely say that it will help keep them manageable. I am sure you have noticed, as I have, that the first sign of bugs or disease is never on your most healthy looking plants. Not at all, but rather you first notice it on your sickly looking plants. When plants are distressed they send out signals that will bring every bug in the area, as well as making them unable to mount any sort of a defense against a virus or blight.

However, the Back to Eden style of gardening will produce the most stress-free environment possible for your plants to grow in. I had mentioned earlier in the book about some volunteer squash that came up through my covering the first year. That squash was always vibrant and healthy looking even in the heat of day. On the other hand, the squash plants in my raised beds would be badly wilted every afternoon and would not regain their normal appearance until the following morning.

Not only did this cause the plant to spend a lot of energy repairing itself after every afternoon (energy that could have been spent growing), but it caused the plants to send out distress signals. That year, for the first time, I had squash bugs in my garden. Guess which plants I found them on first? Yep, it was the sickliest looking ones. In no time at all they were over all the squash plants in my raised beds.

Then, several weeks, later I finally found them on the two huge squash plants growing in the wood chips. I ended up just ripping up all the squash plants early that year to break the lifecycle of the squash bugs, and indeed that worked because I did not see them again the following year. Still, it was a good example of how important it is to have healthy plants to begin with if you want to avoid pest.

The Back to Eden style of gardening provides the healthiest environment possible for the plant. The soil is kept moist, loose, and cool. There is a constant stream of nutrients being washed down by the rains from the decomposing covering overhead. And that same covering dramatically reduces any weeds from stealing those nutrients from the plant.

This all adds up to a wonderful growing environment that will give your plants a fighting chance against bugs and diseases.

Conclusion

Houses are a very important part of our life these days and we really do appreciate and treasure our houses a lot. Houses must be taken good care of and they must also look nice and presentable. If you want to know one way of adding to your house and making it somewhere where you feel at peace you should try working on your backyard.

A yard can make everything seem more connected and more in harmony. If you want a place to relax and be yourself, yo should spend more time creating the perfect and most serene backyard. You will have as much fun creating it as you will spending time in it.

One thing you can add to recreate a sense of growth in your house is to add plants to your garden. Now, you do not have to add flowers because you can do all sort of landscaping techniques with other plants. You can create a dry desert look by growing cacti in your backyard and you will definitely have beautiful flowers on those too. But, if you are a flower type of person you can fill your yard with all sorts of colors and you can establish a safe and beautiful environment. Of course, you can always get colorful plants to do the same thing.

Another thing you can do is add a bird bath or pool in your yard. Bird baths are great because you will get lots of beautiful birds to sing in your house and you will have beautiful yet soft chirping. And you can also install a bird feeder to give the birds and easy way to feast.

Now, if you want a cool place to relax you should consider building a pool. Building a pool is not as hard as everyone thinks it is and you can get this done for a relatively cheap price. So if you want a cool and lively backyard, getting a pool or bird bath is the thing for you.

And if those two are not good options for you, you can always create a patio. Patios are wonderful because you can set up patio furniture and spend time in your back yard relaxing on a comfy sofa of sorts. If you care going to buy patio furniture, you should consider what you are going to put outside. Would you like tables and chairs for your whole family to eat or would you rather have a nice place to lounge? Depending on what you want to have in your backyard you can find lots of cool furniture and styles to buy your stuff in.

After you have set up your backyard you can relax and enjoy the sun shine or the drizzling rain. A backyard is a place to forget all of your worries and escape to a completely different World. If you give yourself the chance to fix up your backyard then you will feel doors open and the breeze come in, literally.

So if you want to create a place for your family to spend time together and relax you can make a home out of a house by fixing up your backyard. Give it a shot, you have nothing to lose at all.

Thank you for purchasing this book, I hope you will apply the acquired knowledge productively.

Would you please be so kind enough to leave a review on Amazon if you have enjoyed this book? It would be highly appreciated. Thanks and good luck!

William Canterbury
http://www.FunHappyLives.com

Made in the USA
Las Vegas, NV
15 April 2024